A Note from the Author

If you enjoyed this book or found it helpful, I would be so grateful if you could take a moment to share your thoughts. Reviews not only support my work but also help others discover resources that may benefit their own wellness journey.

✦ Leave a review on Amazon:
This book was created with AI assistance. While effort has been made to ensure accuracy, the content is for informational purposes only.

★ Or share your feedback on Google:
This book was created with AI assistance. While effort has been made to ensure accuracy, the content is for informational purposes only.

Thank you for being part of the Empower Your Wellness community! Your support means so much.

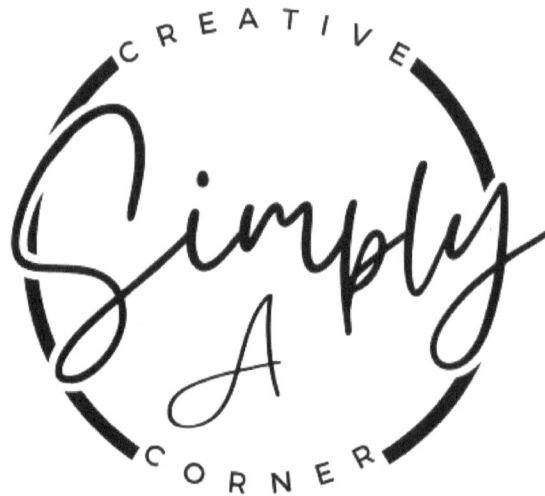

In each corner we use imagination to create

"Welcome to "Herb and Spice Mastery: A Beginner's Comprehensive Guide"! We are delighted to have you embark on this enlightening journey with us. While we may not be experts, we are enthusiastic learners, just like you. Our exploration of the realm of herbs and spices began in the spring of 2023, offering both challenges and rich rewards.

This ebook series was crafted to serve as a complete resource, covering everything you need to know about each herb and spice. Whether you seek quick facts, detailed insights into cultivation, or practical uses, we've got you covered. Remember, we always advise consulting a physician before using any herb or spice for medicinal purposes.

As we progress and acquire more knowledge, we are thrilled to share our discoveries with you through new ebooks. Each edition delves into a different herb, spice, or medicinal plant, expanding our shared knowledge and enriching our well-being together.

Thank you for joining us on this expedition. We hope you derive as much joy and value from these pages as we did in creating them. Let's learn and progress together!"

TABLE OF
CONTENTS

3 BRIEF HISTORY

4 LEGAL NAME, FAMILY, & BOTANICAL

5 HEALTH & MEDICINAL BENEFITS

9 PREPARATIONS & USES & DOSAGE

11 PLANTING

12 GROWING & MAINTENANCE

13 PROPEGATION

14 HARVESTING

15 DRYING & PRESERVING

16 STORING DRIED OREGANO

17 SEED COLLECTION

19 SIDE EFFECTS OR RISKS

20 PESTS & DISEASE

22 UNIVERSAL GUIDELINES

23 HYDROPONICS

25 HERE IS WHAT WE USE

27 SUPPLIES TO GET STARTED-HYDROPONICS

29 ADDITIONAL CONSIDERATION

30 COMPANION PLANTING

32 WHAT WE'VE LEARNED

33 REFERENCES

34 CONTACT US

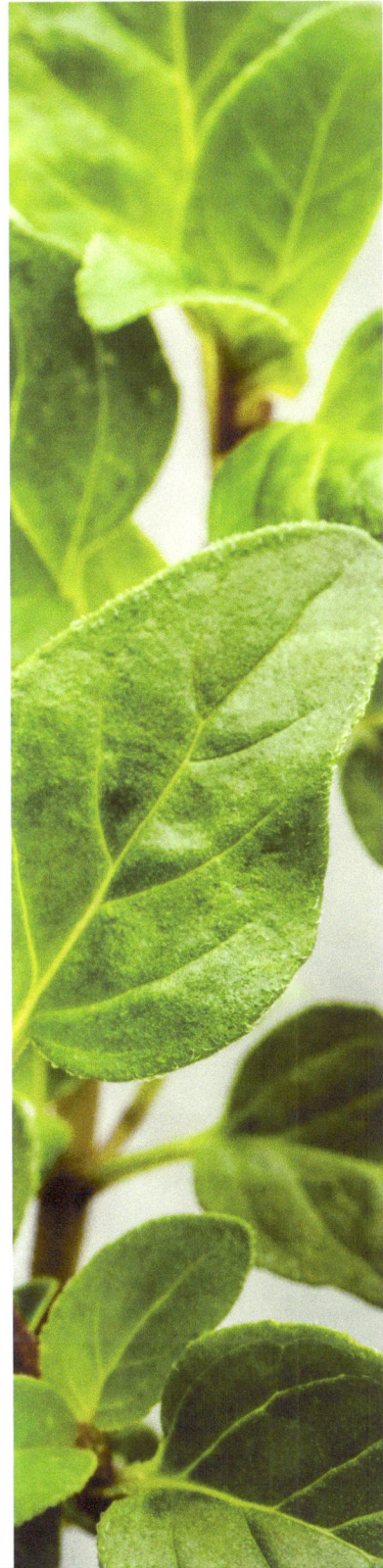

BRIEF HISTORY

The Greeks revered Oregano for its antiseptic, antibacterial, and anti-inflammatory properties. It was often used topically to treat wounds, infections, and skin conditions. Hippocrates, the father of Western medicine, lauded its medicinal benefits and prescribed it for respiratory ailments such as coughs and bronchitis.

the Romans embraced Oregano for its medicinal prowess. They believed in its ability to purify the body and used it to alleviate digestive issues, fevers, and menstrual cramps. The renowned Roman naturalist Pliny the Elder extolled its virtues in his writings, praising it as a panacea for various maladies.

As time progressed, Oregano continued to be valued across cultures and civilizations. In medieval Europe, it was cultivated in monastery gardens and used by herbalists to treat a myriad of ailments, including gastrointestinal disorders and infectious diseases.

During the Renaissance, Oregano's medicinal properties remained highly esteemed. Herbalists like Nicholas Culpeper touted its effectiveness in treating respiratory infections and improving digestion. Oregano was often included in herbal formulations and remedies to combat the prevailing health concerns of the time.

In more recent history, Oregano's medicinal reputation has persisted. With the advent of modern science, researchers have delved into its chemical composition and pharmacological properties. Studies have confirmed its antibacterial, antifungal, and antioxidant activities, lending credence to its traditional uses.

Today, Oregano is a staple in herbal medicine cabinets and kitchen pantries. Its essential oil is prized for its antimicrobial properties and is used in aromatherapy and natural disinfectants. Additionally, Oregano supplements are popular for bolstering immune health and combating infections.

We chose to focus on Oregano due to its abundant and versatile benefits.

3

A

LEGAL NAME

Origanum

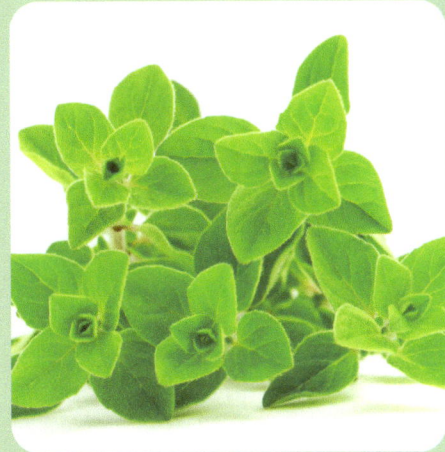

B

FAMILY.

Lamiaceae-Mint Family

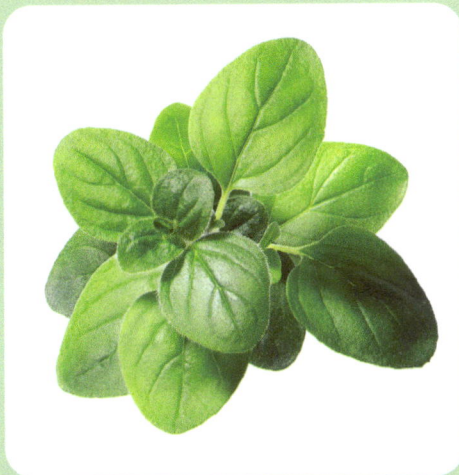

C

BOTANICAL

Perennial herbaceous plant typically grows 18-30 inches high. It has square stems with small, oval-shaped, opposite leaves that are green-gray in color. The leaves are very aromatic and have a strong, spicy flavor. It produces clusters of tiny pick or purple flowers in the summer.

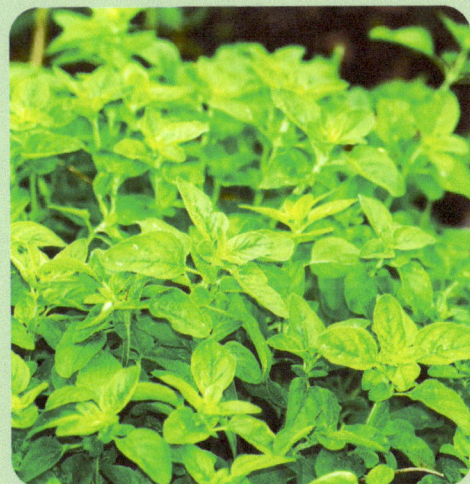

Health & *Medicinal Benefits*

1 Carvacrol

It is a phenol that has demonstrated remarkable antimicrobial activity. This makes oregano a potent ally against various bacterial infections, including those resistant to antibiotics. Its oil, particularly, has been used in folk medicine as a means to combat respiratory ailments, digestive upset, and even skin conditions.

2 Thymol

Is a natural monoterpenoid phenol. Antimicrobial properties fight against bacteria, fungi, and viruses. Reducing the risk of infections and often is used in mouthwashes and hand sanitizers. Antifungal agent is effective in treating fungal infections including those that affect toenails and skin

3 Rosmarinic Acid

- Rosmarinic acid is known for its strong antioxidant effects, which help neutralize harmful free radicals in the body. This can reduce oxidative stress and may help prevent chronic diseases.

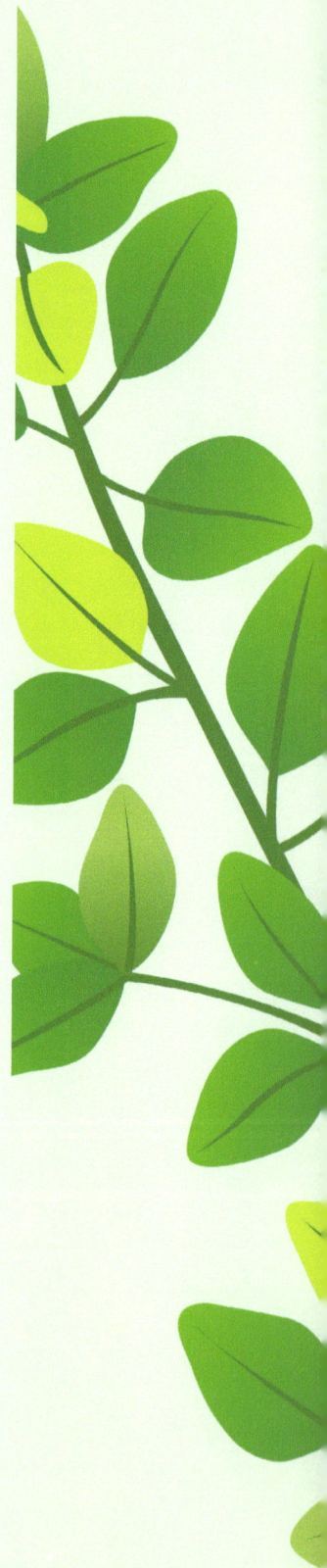

Rosmarinic Acid Cont.

- It has anti-inflammatory properties that make it beneficial for reducing inflammation in various conditions, including asthma, rheumatoid arthritis, and inflammatory allergies.
- Studies suggest that rosmarinic acid may have neuroprotective effects, potentially beneficial in conditions like Alzheimer's disease and other neurodegenerative disorders.
- Rosmarinic acid shows activity against some bacteria and viruses, which might make it useful in treating infections and supporting the immune system.
- Rosmarinic acid is also used in skincare products to help soothe the skin and reduce signs of aging.
-

The compound might help improve cardiovascular health by reducing blood pressure and having antithrombotic effects, which can reduce the risk of clots.

4 Flavonoids

1. Flavonoids are powerful antioxidants, which help neutralize free radicals in the body. This can reduce oxidative stress and may help prevent chronic diseases such as heart disease, diabetes, and cancer.
2. Many flavonoids have strong anti-inflammatory properties. They can help reduce inflammation in the body, which is beneficial for conditions like arthritis, cardiovascular diseases, and even certain neurological conditions.
3. Flavonoids are associated with a reduced risk of cardiovascular disease. They help improve blood vessel function, reduce blood pressure, and decrease LDL cholesterol oxidation.

Flavonoids Cont

4. Rosmarinic acid shows activity against some bacteria and viruses, which might make it useful in treating infections and supporting the immune system.

5. Rosmarinic acid is also used in skincare products to help soothe the skin and reduce signs of aging.

The compound might help improve cardiovascular health by reducing blood pressure and having antithrombotic effects, which can reduce the risk of clots.

5 Terpenes

1. Terpenes are major components in essential oils derived from plants and are often used in aromatherapy, perfumery, and as flavoring agents in foods and beverages.

2. Many terpenes have been shown to have anti-inflammatory effects, which can help treat conditions like arthritis and may contribute to the relief of other inflammation-related conditions.

3. Some terpenes possess antibacterial and antifungal properties, making them useful in reducing infections and as natural preservatives in cosmetics and food products.

4. Certain terpenes, such as linalool (found in lavender) and limonene (found in citrus), are known for their ability to reduce anxiety and stress levels. They are commonly used in stress relief and relaxation products.

5. Terpenes like myrcene, which is found in mangoes and hops, are noted for their analgesic, or pain-relieving properties. They may help alleviate pain and improve comfort.

Terpenes cont

6. Some terpenes may have anticancer properties. For instance, limonene has shown potential in studies to inhibit the growth of cancer cells.
7. Certain terpenes are being researched for their neuroprotective effects, which help in the treatment of neurodegenerative diseases like Alzheimer's and Parkinson's.

In topical applications, some terpenes can enhance the penetration of other active compounds into the skin, making them useful in pharmaceuticals and skincare products.

Preparations, *Uses & Dosages*

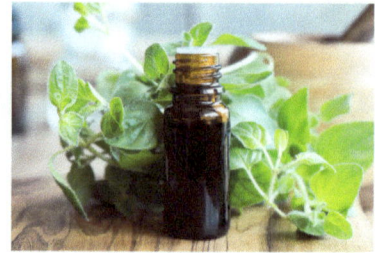

Infusions (Herbal Teas)

Steep 1-2 teaspoons of dried oregano leaves in a cup of boiling water for 10 minutes. Strain and enjoy. Uses: Infusions are excellent for mild digestive issues, easing respiratory symptoms, and providing antioxidants for general health. Dosage: Adults can enjoy 1-3 cups daily. For children aged 5 and above, a half-cup to one cup daily is generally considered safe. Pregnant and breastfeeding mothers should avoid strong infusions and limit consumption to one cup every other day or avoid it, given oregano's potent effects.

Decoctions

Simmer one tablespoon of dried oregano in a pint of water for 10-15 minutes. Strain before use. Uses: Decoctions are more potent than infusions and are beneficial for more severe respiratory issues and infections due to their concentrated form. Dosage: Adults may take up to one cup, twice daily. Not recommended for children, pregnant, or breastfeeding women due to its potency.

Tinctures

Soak dried oregano in a mixture of alcohol and water (40-60% alcohol) for 4-6 weeks, shaking the container daily. Strain the liquid. Uses: Tinctures are used for their antimicrobial properties and to support the immune system. They're particularly effective when taken at the onset of cold or flu symptoms. Dosage: For adults, 2-4 ml three times a day. Not suitable for children, pregnant, or breastfeeding women.

Poultices

Crush fresh oregano leaves and mix with a little hot water to form a paste. Apply directly to the affected area. Uses: Poultices are excellent for skin conditions, bites, and wounds, due to their direct anti-inflammatory and antibacterial properties. Dosage: Can be applied to the skin of adults and children. Use with caution on sensitive skin and avoid in pregnant or breastfeeding women due to potential skin sensitivity.

Salves andOintments

Infuse oregano in a carrier oil (like olive or coconut oil), then mix with beeswax to thicken. Uses: Ideal for fungal skin infections, psoriasis, eczema, and other skin issues. The soothing base also moisturizes the skin. Dosage: Apply topically as needed. Generally safe for adults, children, and breastfeeding mothers if used on small areas of skin. Pregnant women should use with caution and consult a healthcare provider.

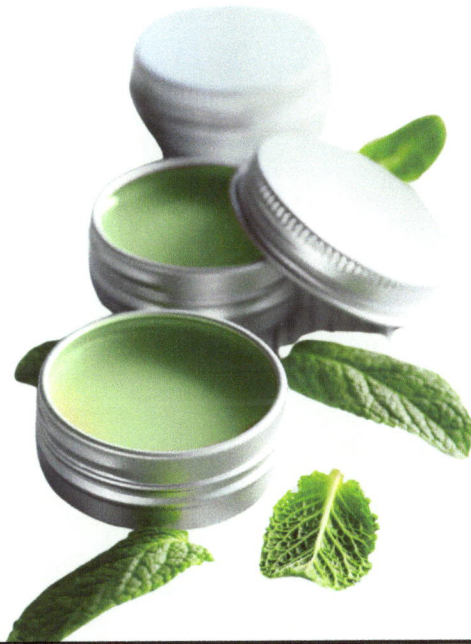

Planting

Select high-quality, organic oregano seeds to ensure a healthy start. Oregano varieties are plentiful, so consider your climate and culinary preferences when choosing.

1. BESTTIME TO PLANT

InfoOregano seeds are best started indoors 6-10 weeks before the last frost date. This herb thrives in warmth, so timing is crucial to avoid cold damage.

2. SOIL PREPARATION

Use a light, well-draining seed starting mix. Oregano prefers a slightly alkaline soil pH, around 6.5 to 7.0. Ensure the soil is moist but not waterlogged.

3. SOWING

Oregano seeds are minuscule, so sprinkle them lightly on the soil surface. Press them gently into the mix without covering them, as they need light to germinate.

4. LIGHT AND TEMPERATURE

Place the seed trays in a warm spot (around 70°F or 21°C) with abundant indirect light or under a grow light. Consistent warmth is key to germination.

5. WATERING NEEDS

Keep the soil consistently moist but not drenched. A spray bottle can moisten the surface without disturbing the seeds.

6. SEED GERMINATION

Expect sprouts in 7-14 days. Once seedlings appear, ensure they receive 6-8 hours of light daily.

Growing &
Maintenance

01. Spacing

When planting oregano, space the plants 8 to 10 inches apart to allow for air circulation and prevent overcrowding, which can lead to disease.

02. Temperatures sunlight req

Oregano thrives in full sunlight. It requires at least 6 to 8 hours of direct sunlight daily. Without adequate sunlight, it may become leggy and produce fewer flavorful leaves.

03. Soil & PH levels

Oregano prefers well-drained, slightly alkaline soil a ph level of 6-8 with good drainage. Sandy or loamy soil types are ideal. However, growing in hydroponics your ph should be slightly lower 5.5 to 6.5 , which helps to ensure absorbsion of nutrients

04. Watering Needs

Water oregano deeply but infrequently, allowing the soil to dry out between watering. Overwatering can lead to root rot.

05. Care & Maintenance

Pruning-Regular harvesting or pinching off the tips encourages bushier growth. Before flowering, oregano's flavor is most potent.

06. Fertilization

Oregano thrives in poorer soils, and too much fertilizer can dilute its flavor. If necessary, use a balanced, organic fertilizer sparingly.

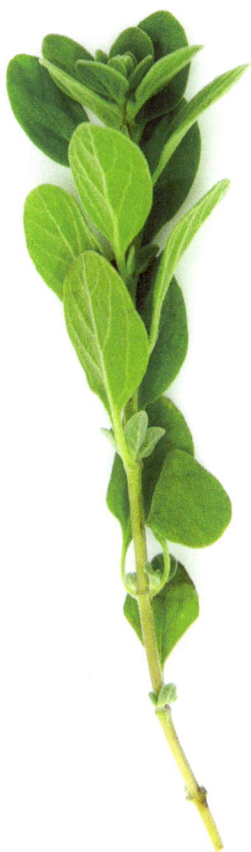

Propagation

01. Cuttings

In late spring or early summer, take 4-6 inch cuttings from healthy, non-flowering stems. Remove the lower leaves and plant the cuttings in moist soil or water until roots develop. This method ensures a true copy of the parent plant.

02. Divisions

InMature oregano plants can be divided in spring or fall. Carefully dig up the plant, ensuring a good root ball. Divide the plant into smaller sections, each with roots and shoots. Replant immediately and water well.fo

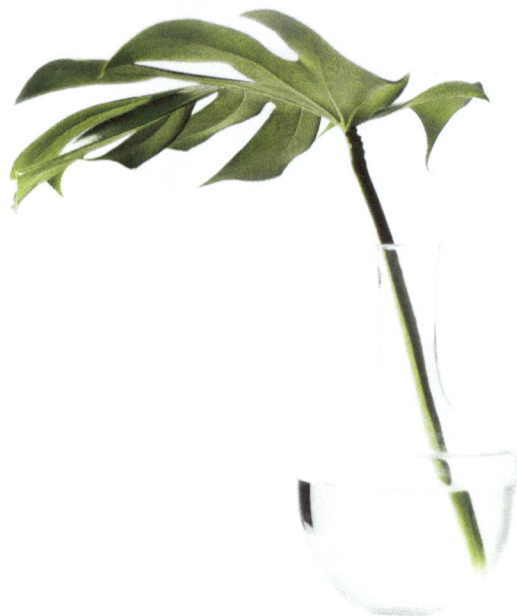

Harvesting

Right time to Harvest

Oregano reaches its peak of flavor and medicinal potency just before it flowers, when the oils in the leaves are most concentrated. Harvesting in the morning after the dew has evaporated but before the sun is high ensures that the essential oils are at their strongest. Look for vibrant, green leaves, signs that the plant is ready to share its bounty.

Harvesting Technique

Trim the stems using clean, sharp scissors or pruning shears just above a leaf node or junction. This allows the plant to regenerate and sustain its growth. Choose healthy stems, steering clear of any that are discolored or damaged. When harvesting, be careful not to take more than one-third of the plant at a time to promote its ongoing health and growth.

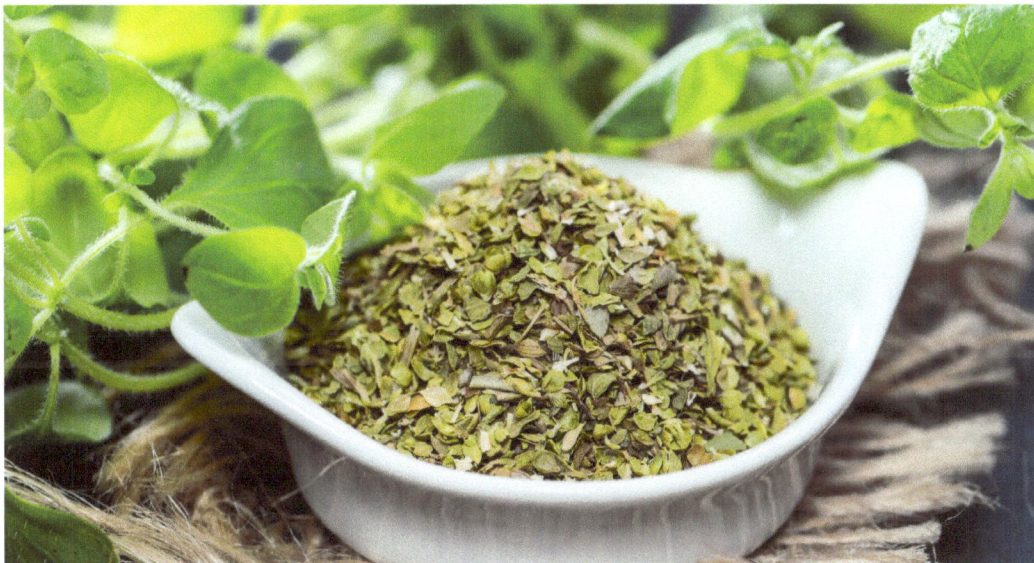

Drying & *Preseving*

Drying is a transformative process, concentrating the herb's flavors and medicinal compounds, and making it shelf-stable for future use.

Drying

Preparation

After harvesting, gently rinse the oregano under cool water to remove any dust or insects. Pat the stems dry with a clean towel or let them air dry on a rack for a few hours.

Bundling

Tie small bunches of oregano stems together with twine or string. Keep the bundles modest in size to ensure even air circulation.

Hanging to Dry

Hang the bundles in a warm, dry, and well-ventilated area out of direct sunlight. Attics, pantries, or even a kitchen can serve as suitable drying spaces. The process can take 1-2 weeks, depending on the humidity and air circulation. The leaves are ready when they are crispy and crumble easily to the touch.

Oven Drying

For a quicker method, oregano can be dried in an oven on the lowest setting. Spread the leaves on a baking sheet and leave the door ajar to allow moisture to escape. Check frequently to prevent burning. This method can dry oregano in a matter of hours.

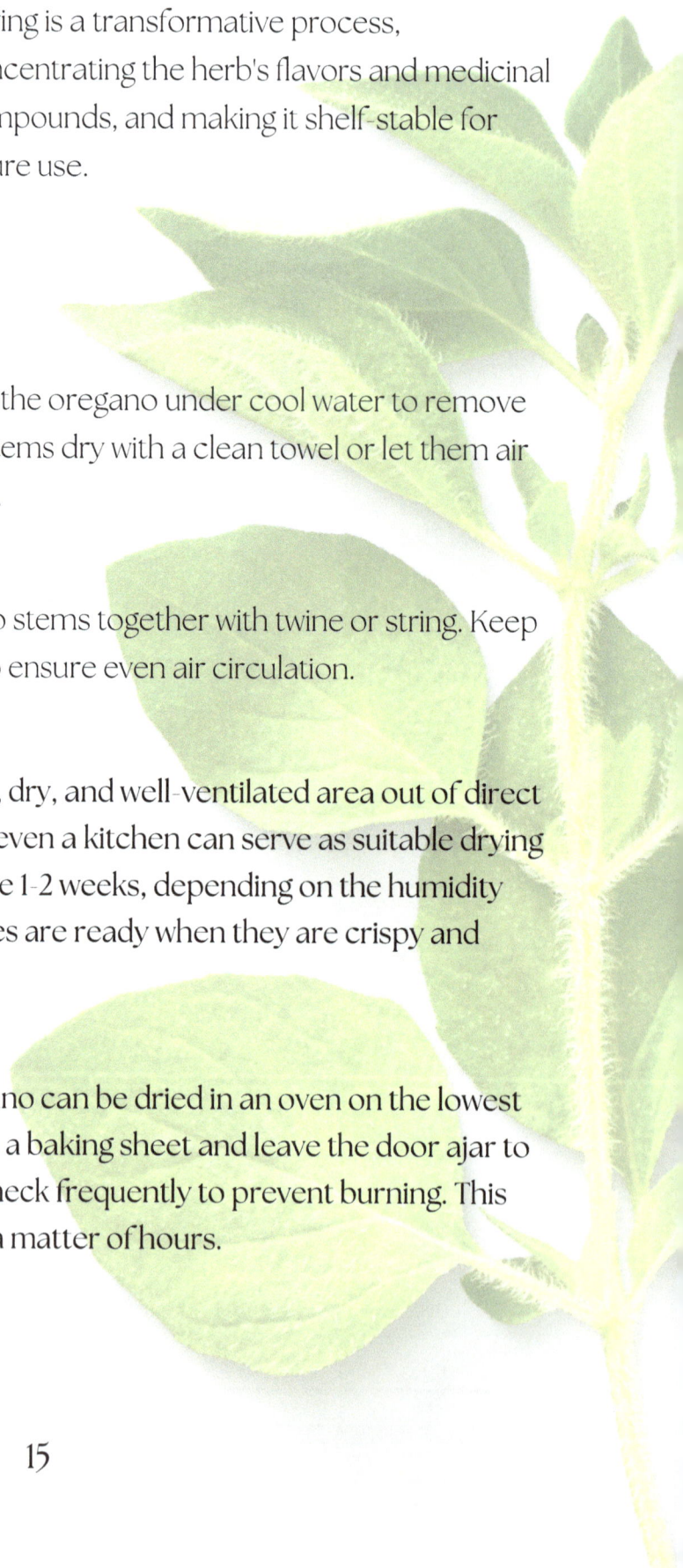

Dehydrator

If you have a dehydrator, it offers the most controlled method for drying herbs. Spread the leaves on dehydrator trays and set the temperature to 95-115°F (35-46°C). The drying time can vary from 1-4 hours.

Storing Dried (Spice)

Once dried, strip the leaves from the stems and discard the stems. Crushing the leaves at this stage can lead to loss of flavor, so it's best to store them whole.

• Airtight Containers: Transfer the dried leaves to airtight containers, such as glass jars with tight-fitting lids. Label the jars with the date of harvest.

• Cool, Dark Place: Store the jars in a cool, dark place like a pantry or cupboard, away from direct sunlight and heat sources, which can degrade the herb's quality.

• Shelf Life: Properly dried and stored oregano can retain its potency for up to a year. After this time, it may lose some of its flavors and medicinal qualities but is still safe to use.

Seed Collection & *Storing*

When to collect Seeds

Oregano seeds in late summer to early autumn. wait until the oregano flowers have bloomed and faded, and the seed heads have begun to dry on the plant. These seed heads will turn a beige or light brown, signaling that the seeds within are ripe and ready for harvest. The ideal time for collection is on a dry day, after the morning dew has evaporated but before the warmth of the day has fully set in.

Collecting the Seeds

- Gather Supplies: You will need a clean, dry container or bag to hold the seeds, and scissors or pruners for cutting.
- Cutting Seed Heads: Carefully cut the seed heads from the plant, taking care to disturb them as little as possible to prevent seeds from falling to the ground.
- Drying: Although the seed heads may appear dry, additional drying ensures that the seeds are fully dry before storage. Place the seed heads in a warm, dry, well-ventilated area on a clean surface or hung in a mesh bag. This process may take a week or more, depending on the humidity levels in your area.
- Extracting Seeds: Once the seed heads are completely dry, gently rub them between your hands over a clean, dry bowl or tray to release the seeds. The seeds are small and may be mixed with chaff.

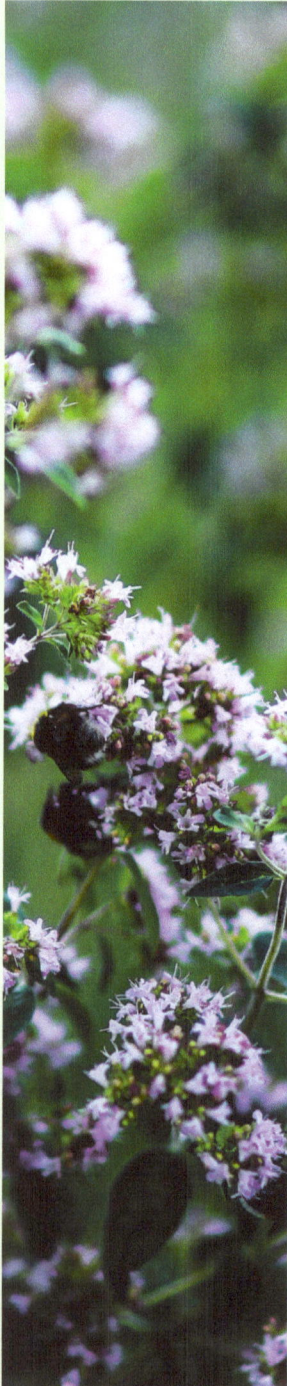

17

- Cleaning: To separate the seeds from the chaff, you can gently blow on the collected material or use a fine sieve that allows the seeds to pass through while catching larger pieces.

Storing Seeds

Proper storage is critical to preserving the vitality of the seeds for future planting. The key factors in storing seeds are cool temperatures, low humidity, and darkness.

- Preparation for Storage: Ensure the seeds are completely dry to prevent mold growth. Any moisture can drastically reduce the viability of the seeds.
- Containers: Use airtight containers for storage, such as glass jars with tight-fitting lids, or sealed plastic bags. Label each container with the seed type and the date of collection.
- Cool, Dark Location: Store the containers in a cool, dark place. A refrigerator is ideal for long-term storage, but a cool pantry or cupboard away from direct sunlight and heat sources works well for shorter periods.

Viability: Properly stored oregano seeds can remain viable for up to 3 years, though it's best to test germination rates if seeds are stored for longer periods by planting a few seeds to see how well they sprout.

Potential Side Effects
Or Risks

> While herbs offer tremendous benefits, they also come with potential side effects or risks, especially when not used judiciously.

Interactions with Medications:

Oregano, particularly in its concentrated oil form, can interact with certain medications, including anticoagulants and diabetes medications. It's essential to consult with a healthcare provider before using oregano medicinally, especially for those on medication.

Allergies and Sensitivities:

Some individuals may be allergic or sensitive to oregano. Patch tests for topical use and starting with small internal doses can help mitigate adverse reactions.

Pregnancy and Breastfeeding:

Due to its potent nature, pregnant and breastfeeding women should use oregano cautiously, particularly the essential oil, as it can affect hormone levels and potentially stimulate the uterus.

Dosage and Concentration:

The adage "the dose makes the poison" holds true for herbal medicine. Even beneficial herbs can become harmful in excessive amounts. It's vital to adhere to recommended dosages and to understand the concentration levels, especially with extracts and oils.

Pests & Disease

In the lush realm of herb cultivation, oregano stands out for its resilience and hardiness. However, like all plants, it is not entirely immune to the challenges posed by pests and diseases.

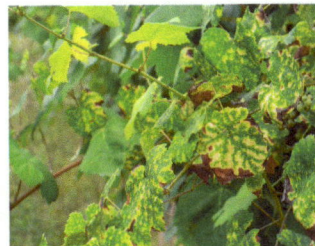

Pests

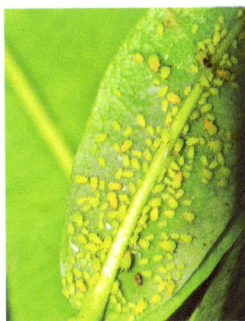

01. Aphids-

These tiny pests sap the life from oregano plants by sucking on the sap of young shoots and leaves, causing them to become distorted and weakened. A strong jet of water can dislodge aphids from your plants. For a more persistent problem, a mild soap solution or neem oil can be applied to affected areas.

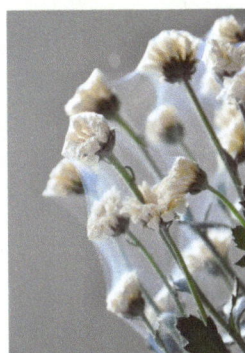

02. Spider Mites

Indicated by fine webbing on the underside of leaves and stunted growth, spider mites thrive in dry conditions. Increase humidity around your plants and use neem oil or a soap solution to treat infestations.

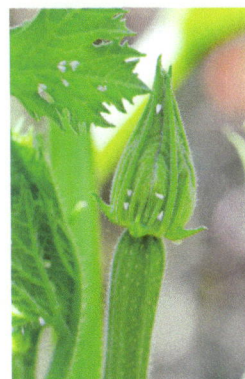

03. Whiteflies

These small, winged pests cluster on the undersides of leaves, sucking sap and weakening the plant. They can be managed by introducing natural predators like ladybugs or by using yellow sticky traps to catch the adults. Neem oil sprays can also reduce whitefly populations.

Diseases

01. Powdery Mildew

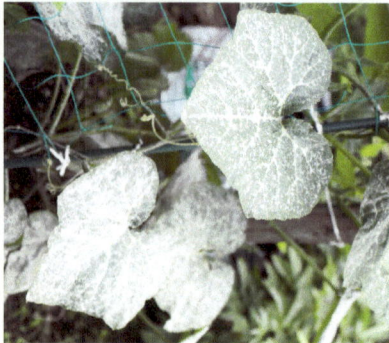

This fungal disease appears as a white powdery coating on leaves and stems, especially during dry, humid conditions. Improve air circulation around your plants and reduce overhead watering to minimize the conditions that favor its spread. Milk spray, a mixture of milk and water, can act as an effective fungicide when applied at the first signs of infection.

02. Root Rot

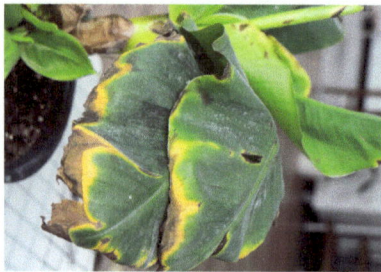

Overwatering is the primary cause of root rot, where the roots of the oregano plant begin to decay, leading to wilting and death. Ensure well-draining soil and moderate watering practices. Infected plants should be removed to prevent the spread of the disease.

03. Botrytis Blight (Gray Mold)

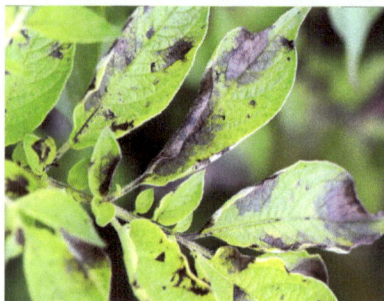

This fungus causes gray, fuzzy mold on leaves, stems, and flowers, thriving in cool, wet conditions. Good air circulation, proper plant spacing, and avoiding wetting the foliage can help prevent botrytis. Remove and destroy infected plant parts at the first sign of disease.

To reduce pests and diseases:
- Remove dead foliage regularly.
- Space out oregano plants for air circulation.
- Plant oregano with tomatoes for health and pest-repellent benefits.
- Attract beneficial insects like ladybugs for pest control and ecological balance.

Universal *Guidelines*

- Adults: Can generally utilize all forms of oregano preparation within recommended dosages.
- Children: Best to stick with milder forms like infusions in reduced strength and quantity. Tinctures and strong decoctions should be avoided.
- Pregnant Women: Caution is advised due to the risk of stimulating the uterus. Infusions should be weak and infrequent if consumed at all. Consultation with a healthcare provider is recommended.
- Breastfeeding Mothers: Limited use of infusions is considered safer, but it's best to consult a healthcare provider. Strong preparations should be avoided to prevent passing of potent compounds to the baby.

Moderation is crucial in all aspects, and understanding one's body and its responses is essential. Herbal remedies, though gentle and natural, are potent aids in maintaining health and should be treated with care. It is advisable to seek advice from a healthcare provider or a skilled herbalist, particularly during pregnancy, while breastfeeding, or when tending to young children, to guarantee the safety and effectiveness of herbal therapies.

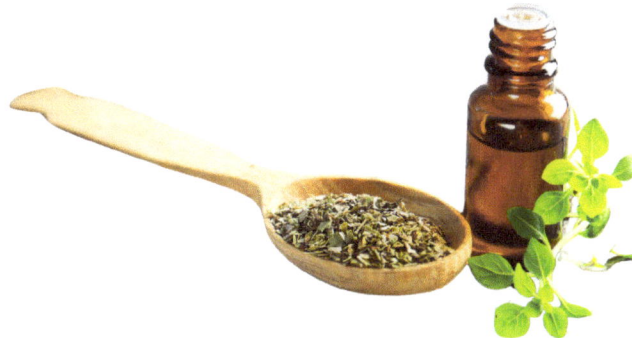

Hydroponics

Hydroponics is a way of growing plants without soil. There are several systems that you can use, with a wide range of cost.

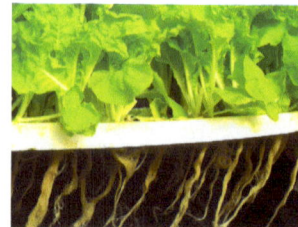

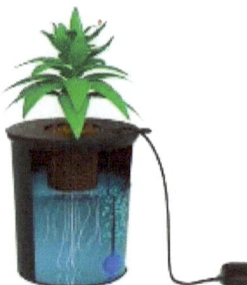

1. DEEP WATER CULTURE (DWC)-PLANT ROOTS ARE SUSPENDED IN A NUTRIENT SOLUTION RESERVOIR. AN AIR PUMP PROVIDES OXYGEN TO THE ROOTS. DWC SYSTEMS ARE RELATIVELY SIMPLE AND INEXPENSIVE TO SET UP, MAKING THEM SUITABLE FOR BEGINNERS. THEY REQUIRE MINIMAL EQUIPMENT AND MAINTENANCE.

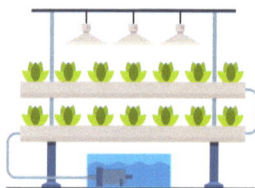

2. NUTRIENT FILM TECHNIQUE (NFT)-INVOLVES A CONTINUOUS FLOW OF NUTRIENT SOLUTION ALONG A SHALLOW, SLOPPING CHANNEL WHERE PLANT ROOTS ARE SUSPENDED. EXCESS SOLUTION IS RECIRCULATED BACK TO THE RESERVOIR. NFT SYSTEMS ARE EFFICIENT IN WATER AND NUTRIENT USAGE BUT MAY BE SLIGHTLY MORE COMPLEX AND EXPENSIVE TO SET UP COMPARED TO DWC SYSTEMS.

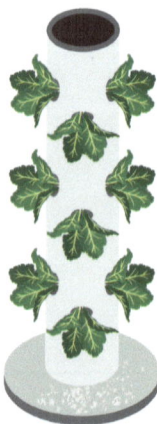

3. DRIP SYSTEM DELIVER NUTRIENT SOLUTION DIRECTLY TO THE PLANT'S ROOT ZONE THROUGH A DRIP EMITTERS OR TUBING. THEY ARE VERSATILE AND CAN BE AUTOMATED FOR PRECISE NUTRIENT DELIVERY. DRIP SYSTEMS CAN VARY IN COMPLEXITY AND COST DEPENDING ON THE SETUP BUT GENERALLY REQUIRE MORE INITIAL INVESTMENT COMPARED TO DWC OR NFT SYSTEMS.

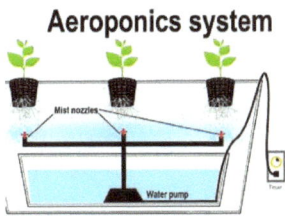
Aeroponics system

4. AEROPONICS SYSTEMS SUSPEND PLANT ROOTS IN THE AIR, AND NUTRIENT SOLUTIONS IS DELIVERED TO THEM AS A FINE MIST OR AEROSOL. THEY ARE HIGHLY EFFICIENT IN WATER AND NUTRIENT USAGE AND CAN PRODUCE RAPID PLANT GROWTH. THEY ARE MORE COMPLEX AND EXPENSIVE TO SET UP AND REQUIRE MORE MAINTENANCE.

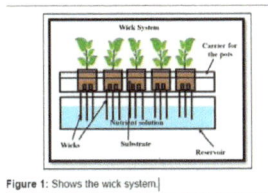
Figure 1: Shows the wick system.

5. THE WICKING SYSTEM USE A WICK TO PASSIVELY TRANSPORT NUTRIENT SOLUTION FROM A RESERVOIR TO THE PLANT ROOTS. THEY ARE SIMPLE AND LOW-COST BUT MAY NOT BE SUITABLE FOR LARGER OR HIGH-WATER DEMAND PLANTS. THIS SYSTEM IS BEST SUITED FOR SMALLER SCALE HOBBYIST SETUPS.

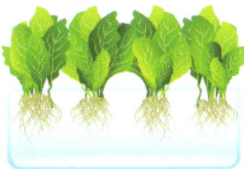

6. THE KRATKY METHOD IS A PASSIVE HYDROPONIC SYSTEM THAT REQUIRES NO ELECTRICITY OR MOVING PARTS. PLANTS ARE PLACED IN A CONTAINER FILLED WITH A NUTRIENT SOLUTION, AND AS THE PLANTS ABSORB THE SOLUTION THE WATER LEVEL DECREASES. THE ROOTS ARE EXPOSED TO BOTH WATER AND AIR, CREATING A BALANCE OF OXYGEN AND NUTRIENTS. THIS METHOD IS STRAIGHT FORWARD AND INEXPENSIVE TO SET UP, MAKING IT AN EXCELLENT CHOICE FOR BEGINNERS OR THOSE WITH LIMITED RESOURCES.

Here is what
We Use

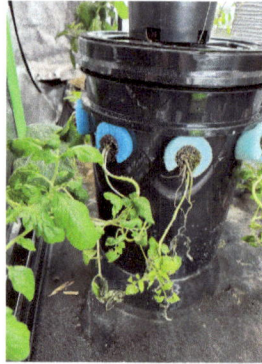

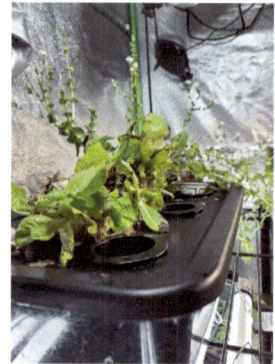

01. Kratky system

We are currently utilizing two different Kratky Systems:

1. Initially, I opted for dish pans with lids and 2" wide-rim net cups. I am opting for shallow containers to avoid excessive depth because I placed them on shelves and connected lights underneath for more space. , I chose black to minimize algae growth, which has been effective. The wide rim of the net cup secures larger plants like lettuce efficiently, yielding up to 8 plants simultaneously. I stagger the plantings to ensure a continuous harvest, starting them in a tray to establish long roots reaching the water while allowing air access.

2. The second system I am exploring is the bucket Kratky system for growing larger plants such as tomatoes and cucumbers. Seeking sturdier support for trellising, I employ black coloration for algae control. Using pool noodles cut into 1.5" sections with a slit for plant roots, I stack the buckets to create a semi-tower setup. Experimenting with different lighting configurations, I am transitioning to tall stand grow lights on four sides for improved growth. Initially starting tomato plants in a tray to establish water-reaching roots, I have one bucket dedicated to tomatoes and plan to set up another for cucumbers. Adapting the nutrient formula for each plant in individual buckets offers flexibility and customization.

02. Drip system

My favorite system is the Farmstead, but it costs steeply. It's not a bad price when you use it outside, but I wanted to grow all winter long so I have mine inside, which means I got the one with lights. Love... love... love this system. It only takes a week or two and you can start harvesting lettuce.

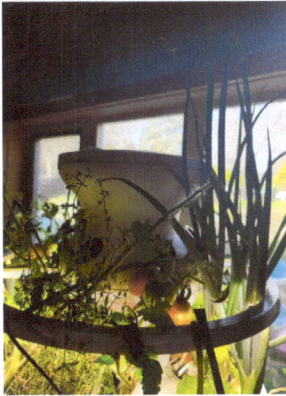

It took a little longer but we have Roma tomatoes growing inside during the winter.

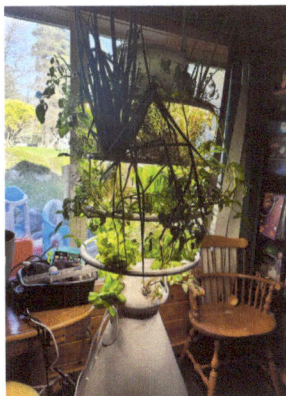

Just look at the growth you can do indoors. I find the system hard to clean, so I will try a different system with a smaller base to see how that works.

Starters

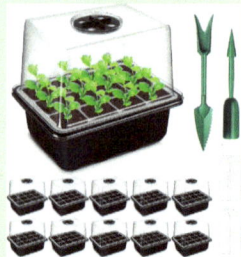

Seed starting trays

https://amzn.to/3xEk6cy

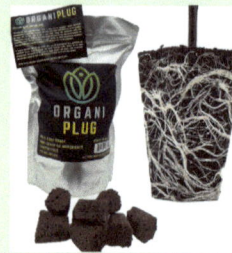

Seed starter Plug

https://amzn.to/4d8eN5m

Heavy Duty Net Pots

https://amzn.to/3W9TVVo

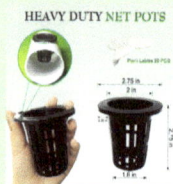

or

Pool Noodles- Use instead of net cups

https://amzn.to/3JsuTJw

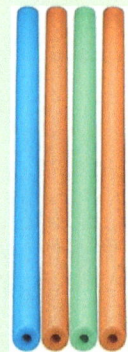

Containers that I use

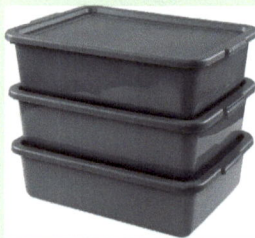

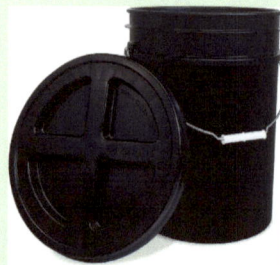

For cutting 2: hole

https://amzn.to/3UpxZnS

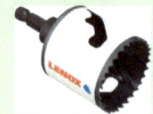

Dish pan for lettuce and spices

https://amzn.to/4d9bOdd

Sturdy buckets for- tomatoes and cucumbers

https://amzn.to/3U6OxBE

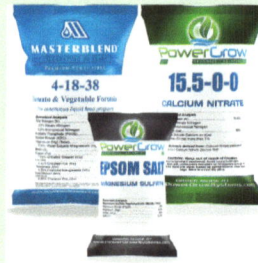

Food

Master Blend Combo Kit

https://amzn.to/3JnPKhj

Lighting

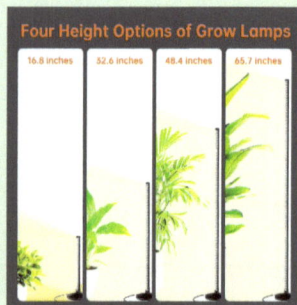

Tall stand lights when you stack your buckets

https://amzn.to/3JnPKhj

Lighting for starter tray and dish trays

https://amzn.to/3WcHFnj

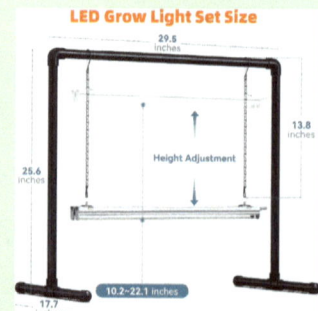

EXTRA'S YOU MAY WANT

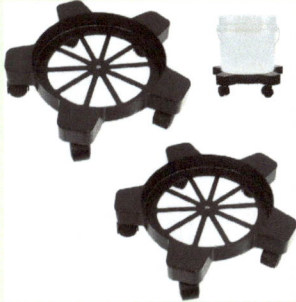

Kennel tray to put everything on. Easy clean up

https://amzn.to/3JsuTJw

Bucket dollies to help you move things around

https://amzn.to/3W76lyt

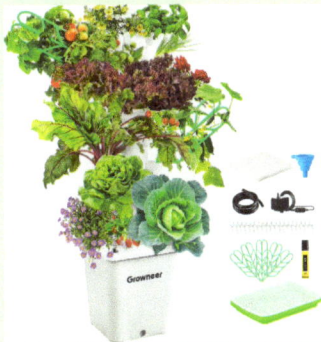

36 plant drip system w/everything including lights

https://amzn.to/49RSLB8

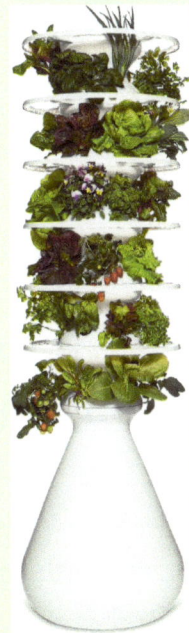

35 plant drip system w/everything no lights

https://amzn.to/3vXdp55

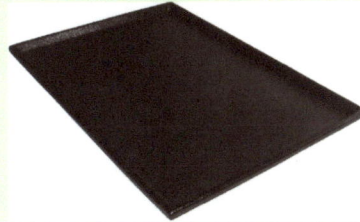

New Lights I found
https://amzn.to/4bp6pfX

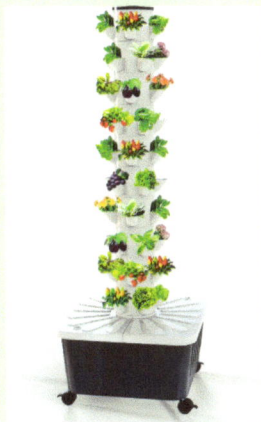

New drip tower I am using
https://amzn.to/3W5qQu1

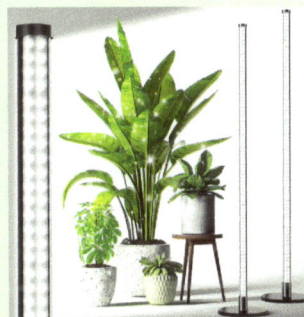

Additional
Considerations

Legal & Ethical

Sustainable Harvesting:
Sustainable practices are paramount whether foraging in the wild or cultivating in gardens. It's essential to harvest in a manner that ensures plants can regenerate, maintaining the health of the ecosystem. This includes taking only what you need and leaving enough behind for the plant to thrive and for wildlife to benefit.

Legal Permissions:
When foraging, be aware of local regulations and property rights. Many areas protect certain species or ecosystems, and foraging without permission can be illegal and harmful to the environment. Please always seek permission from landowners or follow public land guidelines.

Endangered Species:
Some plants are protected due to their endangered status. Herbalists must stay informed about these species to avoid contributing to their decline. Organizations like United Plant Savers provide resources to identify and protect at-risk plants.

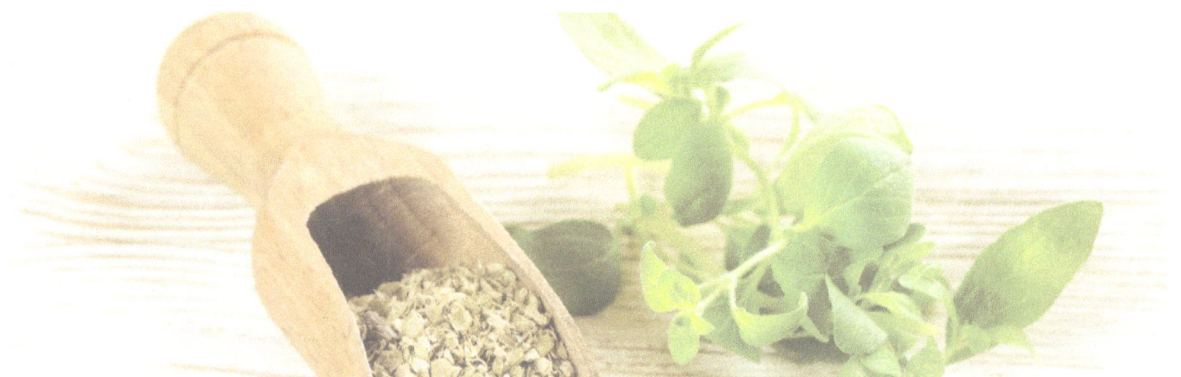

Companion
Planting

spice/herb is a versatile herb that complements many plants when used as a companion. When companion planting, consider the growth habits, sunlight requirements, and soil preferences of each plant to ensure they thrive together. Additionally, interplanting herbs and vegetables can help deter pests, attract beneficial insects, and maximize garden space.

Best Companion plants:

Strawberries

Oregano is a great companion for strawberries as it retains moisture, repels pests, and provides nitrogen. Deer and rabbits are deterred by oregano's scent, while its height ensures it won't overshadow strawberry plants.

Rosemary

Consider planting rosemary as a companion to oregano as its scent deters wildlife and insects. They share growing conditions and can be interplanted to protect other plants from pests effectively.

Asparagus

Asparagus seeds need patience to sprout, taking up to 3 years. Planting oregano alongside can protect them from pests. Asparagus can grow rapidly during peak periods, reaching 5 feet. Prune oregano to prevent overshadowing, but once asparagus thrives, it won't be an issue.

Grapes

Consider planting grapes as companion plants for oregano due to their compatibility in sunny, sandy soils. Grapes grow vertically on trellises, leaving space for oregano to spread. Grapes benefit from nitrogen and can be grown with oregano as a nitrogen-fixing alternative in limited space.

Squash

Squash plants are beginner-friendly and productive but susceptible to pests. Oregano is a beneficial companion plant for squash, preventing soil dryness and repelling insects.

Cucumbers

Oregano acts as a natural repellent for pests like caterpillars, pickle worms, and cucumber beetles attracted to cucumber plants. Planting cucumbers near a trellis for climbing helps their growth and provides shade. The nitrogen boost from cucumber plants benefits oregano.

Thyme

Consider using thyme as a companion plant for oregano to retain moisture in your garden. Both plants grow quickly, contribute to soil nutrients, and act as natural pest deterrents. Plant them among vegetable rows or in flower beds to protect plants from insects.

Melons

Melons such as watermelons and cantaloupes require abundant water due to their sprawling stems and expansive root systems. Oregano, with low water needs, complements melons as its shallow roots draw nutrients from the soil surface. Watering deeply once a week benefits both plants: melons get moisture for their deep roots, while oregano acts as a natural mulch, preserving moisture for the melons to absorb.

Peppers

Bell peppers, jalapenos, and other peppers are good companion plants for oregano due to low water needs. Watering weekly is enough. Removing leaves at the base of pepper plants helps oregano grow. Peppers grow fast but attract pests; oregano's scent repels worms, beetles, caterpillars, and flies.

Avoid planting with these

1. Basil   2. Mint   3. Garlic& Onions   4. Fennel

What we learned

We discovered that Oregano is incredibly simple to start from seed and care for. Right now, I'm cultivating it in a hydroponic setup, and it's thriving beyond expectations. Along the way, as I've been working on this eBook, I've picked up some valuable insights. For instance, I've learned the importance of trimming only a third of the plant to prevent stress, its effectiveness in pest control, and its affinity for growing alongside tomatoes. Sharing this knowledge isn't just about helping others understand this herb; it's also about enriching our understanding as we delve deeper into cultivating natural foods for our families.

Refrences:

Healthify:- https://www.gardeningchannel.com/how-to-grow-oregano/

Natural Food Series: - https://www.gardeningchannel.com/how-to-grow-oregano/

McCormick Science Institue: https://www.mccormickscienceinstitute.com/Our-Research/Scientific-Overviews/MSI-Funded-Paper-Potential-Health-Benefits-of-Oregano

Science-Based Medicine: -https://sciencebasedmedicine.org/oil-of-oregano/ Dr.Axe

Encyclopedia Britannica: https://www.britannica.com/plant/oregano

My Mediterranean Garden: https://mymediterraneangarden.com/plants/origanum-vulgare/

The Nutrition Insider: -https://thenutritioninsider.com/wellness/oregano-benefits/

Verywell Fit: -https://www.verywellfit.com/

Gardening Channel: https://www.gardeningchannel.com/how-to-grow-oregano/

Farmers Almanac: https://www.almanac.com/plant/oregano

The Spruce: https://www.thespruce.com/oregano-growing-guide-5189277

Gardening Know How: https://www.gardeningknowhow.com/edible/herbs/oregano/oregano-companion-planting.htm

Home Live to plant: https://livetoplant.com/greek-oregano-plant-soil-how-to-choose-the-right-type/

Eden Green: https://www.edengreen.com/blog-collection/hydroponic-oregano-guide

Gardening Tips: https://gardeningtips.in/growing-oregano-hydroponically-a-full-guide

Thank You from Simply A Creative Corner

From all of us at Simply A Creative Corner, thank you for purchasing this book and being part of the Empower Your Wellness journey. We truly appreciate your support and hope this resource inspires you on your path to natural healing and healthy living.

We'd Love Your Feedback

Your review means the world to us! Reviews not only support our work but also help others discover resources that may improve their wellness journey.

✨ Leave a review on Amazon:
https://www.amazon.com/stores/Melissa-Poehler/author/B0FNS4WPT9?ref=sr_ntt_srch_lnk_1&qid=1758210089&sr=8-1&isDramIntegrated=true&shoppingPortalEnabled=true&ccs_id=61bd26bb-9338-4d61-8b7e-f428c48f7cec

★ Or share your feedback on Google:
https://g.page/r/CUAi1lOaMhXaEAI/review

Need Assistance?

If you have any questions or need support, please contact us at:
◾ CustomerService@SimplyACreativeCorner.com

Stay Connected

Join our Wellness Corner to stay updated with new releases, wellness tips, and special offers:
https://systeme.io/dashboard/share?hash=75143867cd1b9b84a0e32d5f780ef18941e6&type=campaign

Thank you again for your support—together, we're creating a space where imagination, creativity, and wellness meet.